Fibromyalgia

A Guide to Understanding and Managing Fibromyalgia

Table of Contents

Introduction

Have you walked on the road at night with no light source and kicked a stone or hard object, hurting your toe? Have you been in the kitchen slicing some tomatoes and accidentally cut your hand? Have you experienced heartbreak in relationships, or lost someone close to you? If the answer is yes to any of these questions, then you know what pain feels like.

From these scenarios, you can see that there is always a possibility to experience pain in different areas of our life and that it is impossible to live without experiencing pain at one point or another. The pains described above all have expiry periods, as our bodies heal with time, no matter the type of injury, illness, or hurt. Some afflictions might last longer than others; for example, the pain experienced from kicking a stone cannot be compared to the pain of losing a loved one.

In some people, however, the pain does not have an expiry period as they go about their daily routines with pain in every part of their body even if they have not been injured. This is caused by a condition that inhibits the way the body processes pain. This condition is called fibromyalgia and it can occur in people of all ages, walks of life, and locations around the world.

This pain affects the musculoskeletal system and the nervous system, which is responsible for transferring the pain signals to the brain.

Fibromyalgia (FBM) is a chronic disorder that affects all nerve endings due to the body's abnormal pain perception processing. This condition has no cure, but the symptoms can be managed by doctors and other health professionals through medication as well as a variety of alternative treatment methods. This book provides an in-depth analysis of the science that helps explain what's responsible for causing fibromyalgia and how the condition can be managed. Whether you are personally suffering from fibromyalgia, or if you are simply looking to better understand what a loved one is going through, this book will help you to gain a full understanding of what fibromyalgia is, what the symptoms are, and how they can be managed and improved.

Chapter One: What is Fibromyalgia?

Fibromyalgia is an ailment that is marked by extensive pain in the musculoskeletal system of the body. It is characterized by sleep problems, tiredness, memory loss, and constant mood swings. Medical studies have shown that from how the message of pain is interpreted in the brain and spinal cord, fibromyalgia can exasperate this painful stimulation. In other words, the brain cells sometimes respond excessively or misconstrue body pain signals. This can sometimes be because of a disproportion in the brain chemicals or a malfunction in the dorsal root ganglion. When this happens, the pain nerves in the body are severely affected.

Fibromyalgia is a prevalent ailment. In fact, it is the second most common musculoskeletal ailment. It causes not only joint pain and discomfort to the body but can also cause mental stress.

One reason fibromyalgia seems to be a complicated ailment is that it is very difficult to diagnose correctly. Although most medical experts view fibromyalgia as a rheumatic syndrome, there are no actual tests to verify the authenticity of a fibromyalgia diagnosis. Because it may cause soft tissue pain or myofascial pain, many diagnoses mistake fibromyalgia for arthritis. Nevertheless, fibromyalgia differs from arthritis in that it does not show any form of muscular or joint inflammation. Generally, there is no cure for fibromyalgia. It can only be medically managed using a mix of psychological and physiotherapeutic treatment. One who is suffering from fibromyalgia may need to adopt a new healthy lifestyle to live their lives optimally. Thankfully, we are slowly gaining more understanding of fibromyalgia and new treatment methods are being developed over time.

The causes of fibromyalgia are generally known as "regions of pain." These are regions of the body known as tender or trigger points. It has been observed that these regions often overlap with each other. Sometimes, when an individual has suffered from an infection or a traumatic condition or has been through a surgery, or even if they have been stressed psychologically, fibromyalgia symptoms may begin to show. It appears as though as a response to stress on the body, fibromyalgia develops and begins sending pain signals despite there being nothing physically "wrong".

Further studies have shown that men are less likely to suffer from fibromyalgia. Medical researchers have also found that people with fibromyalgia may also suffer from some underlying ailments such as temporomandibular (TMJ) disorders, depression, anxiety, headaches, irritable bowel syndrome, chronic fatigue syndrome, interstitial cystitis, and postural tachycardia syndrome.

Those who are most at risk of fibromyalgia include those with a family history of fibromyalgia. Anyone who has arthritis is also at risk.

Myths About Fibromyalgia

People may not take you seriously when you complain constantly of joint aches and body pain, but this pain is a daily reality for people who have fibromyalgia. Many people around them and even medical practitioners are often quick to dismiss the seriousness of this claim. This dismissal might be because of the indefinite diagnostic nature of fibromyalgia. You have probably heard many things about fibromyalgia, some true, some false, and maybe even some half-truths. The following are some of the myths you may have heard about fibromyalgia:

1. **Fibromyalgia is fake.** Many people all over the world still believe that fibromyalgia is not legitimate. Their reason for this is that fibromyalgia has no real symptoms; it is more of a syndrome. That is, it's a summation of a variety of signs. These symptoms are recorded and diagnosed best by a fibromyalgia specialist.

2. **Anyone can diagnose fibromyalgia**. There is a widespread falsehood that anyone can diagnose fibromyalgia. This is simply not true. A fibromyalgia specialist is the best person to diagnose a fibromyalgia

condition. To diagnose fibromyalgia, a specialist has to investigate the medical history of the sufferer, as well as assess some tender points in their body.

3. **It has a hidden cause.** Some people believe that fibromyalgia is hereditary or a result of someone's geographic locale. Others believe that fibromyalgia could be caused by coalescence. Contrary to the mystical belief of many people, the cause of fibromyalgia is still unknown.

4. **There are no treatments for fibromyalgia.** Although fibromyalgia may not be cured, it can be managed with the help of a medical practitioner. Some of these treatments can help reduce the pain in your body and improve your physical health. Not all of the remedies for treating fibromyalgia come in pill form. In fact, one of the most effective treatments for fibromyalgia is simply to change your lifestyle. The treatment and management of fibromyalgia is usually all-encompassing and will include things such as medication as well as focusing on sleep, diet, exercise, stress-reduction, and more.

5. **All medical practitioners understand fibromyalgia.** Have you ever opened up to your doctor and explained the pain in your body, but they couldn't seem to understand your condition despite your

illustrations and descriptions? This is precisely what people with fibromyalgia go through every day in hospitals, clinics, and in the hands of doctors. Most times, the pain of fibromyalgia is unexplainable. Unfortunately, because of a late diagnosis, the symptoms and effects of fibromyalgia may have settled deep into the musculoskeletal system. Despite the extensive signs, due to the many mysteries surrounding fibromyalgia, many medical practitioners are yet to fathom the true nature of the fibromyalgia ailment.

6. **Fibromyalgia has a generic diagnosis.** There's a perception that fibromyalgia is a fallback diagnosis since laboratory tests are not sufficient or accurate enough to diagnose it, and a physical examination does not make up for this. Fibromyalgia does not have a comprehensive diagnosis; instead, it is usually very directional in its diagnosis.

7. **Fibromyalgia only affects women.** It is false to believe that fibromyalgia is a feminine ailment. Although several kinds of research, reports, and statistics show evidence that fibromyalgia mostly affects women, it can still affect men. The National Fibromyalgia Association (NFA) reported that approximately 3 out of every four diagnosed with fibromyalgia are women.

8. **Fibromyalgia and arthritis are the same.** You may be committing a blunder if you think that fibromyalgia and arthritis are the same musculoskeletal condition. The symptoms may appear similar, but that does not mean that they are the same. There is a slight difference between fibromyalgia and arthritis. While people living with fibromyalgia and arthritis may both experience muscular tiredness and pain, arthritis is also accompanied by inflammation, whereas fibromyalgia involves just the pain and tiredness with no obvious cause.

9. **People with fibromyalgia need to be placed on a diet.** Is fibromyalgia a dietary ailment? No, it isn't. Recent research conducted by the National Institutes of Health (NIH) has shown no dietary remedy for fibromyalgia. However, while it's not a cure, many people do experience a reduction in the severity of their symptoms in response to eating a healthy diet free from alcohol and processed foods.

10. **Alternative remedies are of no use.** Have you tried to alleviate the symptoms of fibromyalgia using alternative remedies such as yoga, qigong, and tai chi? Many of those who have tried these practices have experienced significant changes and improvements in their health as a result. These alternative remedies are

also called meditative movement therapies. Research conducted by Rheumatology International revealed that individuals who correctly applied these alternative remedies experienced improved sleep, and were able to fight depression, tiredness, and anxiety successfully. It was also discovered that a connective tissue massage could help to alleviate fatigue, sleeplessness, and depression, particularly with women suffering from fibromyalgia.

11. **It would be best if you avoid exercise.** Should persons who have fibromyalgia stay away from exercise? Well, until proven otherwise, regular exercise remains the most potent remedy for fibromyalgia. Recent research by the American College of Rheumatology made that discovery. Aerobic exercise such as walking or hiking, jogging or running, biking, swimming, rowing, in-line skating, and skiing have proven to help people living with fibromyalgia get better and recover faster. Another medical study also shows that regular stretching is a good exercise for people with fibromyalgia. Engaging in regular activity as a person with fibromyalgia will come with some difficulty at first, but over time will be a worthwhile endeavor.

12. **It is just a feeling of fatigue.** A lot of people believe that fibromyalgia is just a mere feeling of fatigue. This

may appear to be the case looking from the outside in, but people living with fibromyalgia know that it is not just a feeling but rather something more profound. The level of fatigue fibromyalgia causes is extraordinary and is also accompanied by other symptoms.

13. **People with fibromyalgia are helpless.** There is no known cause of fibromyalgia, and there is no known cure for fibromyalgia. Does this mean that anyone who has fibromyalgia is utterly hopeless? No! Not at all! Numerous medical and alternative treatments can help one ease the symptoms of fibromyalgia. If you have fibromyalgia, you do not need to pigeonhole yourself into one form of treatment. There are many different ways to approach your diagnosis and begin gaining control over your symptoms.

Chapter Two: Potential Causes and Risk Factors of Fibromyalgia

It is normal to get injured at times; these moments are natural parts of life. The body is composed of many systems, organs, tissues, nerves, and cells that serve in different capacities for the body to perform all its functions successfully. A deviation in the performance or an inability of the body to carry out all its functions is referred to as a disease. All cells in the body know the functions they are to perform, and if your body is in good health, these functions are completed like a well-oiled machine.

When you get injured, the cells that are responsible for healing the injury should begin their functions immediately. The first thing the body does is inform us of the pain that comes with getting injured. Information is passed in the body by using nerve signals; there are nerve endings in many areas of the body, and they are responsible for informing the body of different sensations.

Immediately when we get injured, nerve signals travel from the injured area to the brain through the spinal cord. The brain interprets the signal as pain and sends a notification that something is wrong with the body. As the injury heals, the pain decreases and goes away when the wound is fully healed. You should only experience pain when you are injured.

Another way to think of it is to picture the body like a phone that sends you a notification whenever it is close to any open Wi-Fi hotspot. You should only receive notifications when there is an available hotspot; you should not get any Wi-Fi notifications if there are no open Wi-Fi hotspots around.

Fibromyalgia patients typically feel pain all over their bodies even when they are not sick or injured. Unlike pain caused by injuries that goes away when the injury heals, this pain does not go away. Not only will these patients constantly feel pain, but minor wounds and bruises will hurt a lot more than they usually would. They will also feel pain from things that should not cause pain at all.

There are no universally agreed-upon causes of this disease. Some doctors suspect that it is caused by a defect in the way the brain and spinal cord interpret pain signals, though currently, nobody knows for certain.

What we do know universally is that when you have fibromyalgia, it means that you have more cells that carry pain signals to the brain than usual. The increase in the number of pain-carrying signals coincides with a reduction in the cells that are responsible for slowing down pain. When this occurs, the pain never ends, and it is like your pain volume is always turned up regardless of the condition of the body.

Possible Causes for Fibromyalgia

Many people have reported different causes for their condition, so it seems possible to have more than one cause for fibromyalgia. Many things can cause pain signals to go askew. Some of the causes are explained below.

Genetics

Research has been carried out to determine the causes of fibromyalgia, and it has been suggested that genetics can have a part to play in the development of it. Studies have shown that people are more likely to suffer from fibromyalgia if they also have a parent with fibromyalgia, though the exact genes responsible for this are unknown.

Abnormal pain messages

The difficulty the brain has in processing electrical signals has been identified as one of the causes of fibromyalgia. This difficulty that is experienced could be the result of changes to chemicals present in the nervous system. Information should be transferred all over the body by the central nervous system (CNS) using a network of specialized cells, but when there is a change in the workings of the CNS, it causes increased sensitivity to pain and a constant feeling of discomfort. Earlier I mentioned that the causes are relatively unknown and that there are just theories of what they could be. The theory of abnormal pain messages is supported by the fact that most people who have fibromyalgia usually have other medical conditions that affect how the CNS processes pain. Some of these conditions could be migraines, irritable bowel syndrome (IBS), or craniomandibular disorders, which affect the jaw muscles and joints.

Chemical imbalances

I mentioned earlier that the brain is responsible for interpreting the signals that are sent to it from various nerve endings. There are some hormones in your brain that enable it to carry out its functions; if there is a deviation from the optimal level of hormones in the brain, its functions are inhibited. Research has shown that people who have fibromyalgia have low levels of the hormones serotonin, noradrenaline, and dopamine in their brains.

The low levels of these hormones could be a factor as they are responsible for regulating some feelings in the body, such as mood, appetite, sleep, behavior, and response to stress. Dopamine, noradrenaline, and serotonin are also involved in the process of interpreting the pain signals that are sent by the nerves. Studies have also pointed to increased levels of the hormone cortisol, which is released when the body is under stress, as a contributing factor to triggering Fibromyalgia.

Sleep disorders

Disrupted or disturbed sleep patterns are generally classified as one of the symptoms of Fibromyalgia, but it could also be a cause. People suffering from Fibromyalgia indeed find it difficult to sleep deeply, which causes daytime fatigue. People who sleep badly can also suffer from high levels of pain, which suggests that lack of sleep contributes to other symptoms of fibromyalgia.

Risk Factors of Fibromyalgia

Studies have shown that Fibromyalgia can affect different kinds of people living in different locations, from different religions, sexual orientations, genders, and races, but its occurrence has shown to be more common in some people than in others. These factors are explained below:

Gender

Studies have shown that Fibromyalgia is more common in women than men. Doctors presume that the differences in the occurrence of this condition in both genders could be because of the contrasting way that men and women react to pain as well as the societal expectation of reactions to pain.

Lack of exercise

Research has shown that Fibromyalgia has a higher occurrence in people who are not physically active. This theory is supported by the fact that exercise is one of the treatment methods prescribed to people living with the condition.

Emotional and physical abuse

There is a higher chance of children who have experienced abuse developing fibromyalgia when they grow up than those that have not experienced abuse. Studies have shown that abuse affects and changes the way that the body responds to pain and stress.

Post-Traumatic Stress Disorder (PTSD)

Some people develop mental health issues after they have witnessed or lived through a horrible event such as sexual assault, death, war, accidents, or kidnapping. The reaction exhibited due to such circumstances has been linked to the development of fibromyalgia in some people.

Age

There is no age restriction to being diagnosed with this condition. This condition can affect people of all ages, even children. Studies have shown, however, that fibromyalgia is most commonly diagnosed in people during middle age and that the chance of developing fibromyalgia increases as you get older.

Lupus or Rheumatoid Arthritis

Lupus is an autoimmune disease where the immune system that should fight harmful cells from affecting the body starts attacking healthy cells mistakenly. Rheumatoid arthritis (RA) is a kind of arthritis that affects the joints of the body. People who suffer from this condition experience pain, stiffness, and loss of function in the joints. It affects many parts of the body, but it is more common in the wrist and fingers. People who suffer from lupus and rheumatoid arthritis have a higher chance of developing fibromyalgia.

Repetitive injuries

A few pieces of research have suggested a link between repetitive injuries and the development of Fibromyalgia. Injuries that occur as a result of repetitive stress on a joint such as frequent knee bending could potentially increase your chances of developing fibromyalgia.

Infections

The presence of an illness, especially a viral infection, could trigger the development of fibromyalgia or could increase the occurrence of its symptoms. Illnesses such as the flu, pneumonia, gastrointestinal infections caused by salmonella and shigella bacteria, and the Epstein-Barr virus have been linked to fibromyalgia.

Localized recurrent pain

Based on the cases of fibromyalgia that have been reported, several studies have shown that people who experience recurrent pain in a specific part of the body have a higher chance of developing this condition.

Chapter Three: Signs, Symptoms, and Triggers of Fibromyalgia

As noted in the previous chapters, fibromyalgia is a condition that involves general body pain. Some possible causes include fatigue, sleep problems and disorders, mental and emotional distress, genetics, and not moving enough. In this chapter, we'll be exploring some of this condition's common signs and symptoms.

Common Signs and Symptoms of Fibromyalgia

Fibromyalgia causes what's now popularly referred to as *regions of pain*. Some of these regions overlap with what used to be known as areas of tenderness, usually known as *tender points* or *trigger points*. To clarify, some of these areas previously noted as tender points are no longer included. The pain in these areas usually feels like a constant dull ache. Your healthcare practitioner will consider a diagnosis of fibromyalgia if, at least once, you ever experienced musculoskeletal pain in at least four out of the five regions of pain delineated some years ago in the revisions of the fibromyalgia diagnostic criteria.

This diagnostic protocol is known as *multisite pain*. This diagnosis procedure emphasizes the regions of musculoskeletal pain and severity of pain in contrast to focusing on the duration of pain, which was previously the focal point for a fibromyalgia diagnosis.

Findings have shown that fibromyalgia has several symptoms, and they vary from one individual to the next. The main symptom is widespread pain; there may be times when the symptoms get better, and sometimes, worse. Some factors commonly impact the severity of symptoms, such as:

- Weather conditions

- Physical activity

- Stress levels

If you are noticing symptoms of fibromyalgia, it is advised that you book an appointment to see your family doctor, also known as a General Practitioner. A GP may be able to diagnose and treat fibromyalgia but, if not, request a referral to a specialist such as a rheumatologist, osteopath, or neurologist.

Although treatments are available to relieve some of the symptoms, the chances are high that you will not get relief instantly. This is a long-term commitment to discovering and implementing the best course of pain relief for your particular situation. The primary signs of fibromyalgia are listed below:

Widespread pain

Widespread pain is the most famous sign and symptom of fibromyalgia. Once you realize you are having widespread pain through all parts of your body, most especially in particular regions such as your neck or back, there is every possibility that you have fibromyalgia. It is usually a continuous pain, even though you may feel better or worse at different times. The pain could feel like a sharp, stabbing pain, a burning sensation, or an ache.

Rigidity

Fibromyalgia can make you feel rigid. The rigidity might be even worse when you have stayed in a particular position for an extended period. For instance, you may feel such pain immediately after getting out of bed in the morning. Stiffness can make your muscles contract, making them tight and painful.

Oversensitivity

Fibromyalgia can make you oversensitive. You will feel extremely sensitive to pain all over your body and you may discover that you feel injured even at the slightest touch. If you accidentally hurt yourself, maybe by stubbing your toe, you may feel continuous pain for a long time beyond what is considered normal.

Medically, this condition is best described using either of the following terms:

- **Allodynia:** The condition when you feel pain from something that shouldn't have caused you pain at all, e.g., a very light touch.
- **Hyperalgesia:** This is the condition when you're extremely sensitive to pain.

You may also be sensitive to other things like bright lights, smoke, and certain foods. Also, when you get exposed to the stimuli you're sensitive to, it may lead to other symptoms of fibromyalgia emerging.

Sleep disorders

Poor quality of sleep is often described as non-restorative sleep. Fibromyalgia can make your rest take a negative turn. For people with fibromyalgia, there will often be times when you wake up very tired even though you've had enough time to sleep. This is because the condition can sometimes deprive you of quality sleep, thus you won't wake feeling refreshed.

Incessant headaches

Invest time to listen to your body, especially your head; those who do this and discover that they have a headache most of the time may have fibromyalgia. Fibromyalgia commonly makes you experience stiffness and pain in your neck and shoulders region, and this is often accompanied by recurrent headaches. These symptoms take different forms, from having mild headaches to severe migraines, and in some instances, you may feel sick.

Fibro-fog

Fibro-fog and cognitive problems are conditions related to mental processes such as thinking and learning. Any individual who has fibromyalgia may experience some of the following symptoms:

- You may experience difficulty speaking or have slowed or confused speech

- You may find it difficult to remember and learn new things

- You may find it hard to pay attention and focus or concentrate

Irritable Bowel Syndrome (IBS)

Some people with fibromyalgia also develop irritable bowel syndrome (IBS). IBS is a common digestive ailment that causes pain and bloating in your stomach. It can lead to inflammatory bowel diseases such as diarrhea or constipation.

Fatigue

Fibromyalgia can cause fatigue or extreme tiredness. This can vary from a mild tired feeling to the overtiredness often experienced with flu-like dizziness. Extreme weariness may suddenly occur and can drain you of all your energy.

Depression

Studies have shown that in some cases, fibromyalgia can lead to depression. This is primarily because of how frustrating and debilitating fibromyalgia can be. In addition, low levels of chemicals in the brain such as serotonin can be a contributing factor. Symptoms of depression include:

- Constantly feeling helpless and hopeless

- Not having an interest in the things you used to enjoy doing

- Feeling low and constantly unmotivated

If you are experiencing depression, it would be best to seek medical attention from a GP, psychologist, psychiatrist, or a fibromyalgia healthcare expert.

Other symptoms of Fibromyalgia

Other symptoms that individuals with fibromyalgia sometimes experience include:

- Anxiety

- Dry eyes

- Restless legs syndrome

- Dull ache in the lower gut or a stabbing pain

- Interstitial cystitis

- Unusual painful periods

- Feeling too hot or cold: inability to regulate body temperature properly

- Inability to stay focused or pay attention

- Numbness, prickling, tingling, or burning sensations in your hands and feet (pins and needles, also known as paresthesia)

- Lack of energy

- Memory problems

- Muscle cramps or twitches

- Burning, itching, and other skin related issues

Most Severe Symptoms

As rightly noted, fibromyalgia can make you feel intense and constant pain. It can be so debilitating that it keeps you from engaging in your day-to-day activities. It might even leave you with no choice but to stay at home. In a National Health Interview Survey, 87% of participants reported pain on most or all of their days. It has been noted that fatigue can have the most impact on an individual's life out of all the fibromyalgia symptoms. Research shows that constant fatigue affects more than 90% of people with fibromyalgia.

Fibromyalgia fatigue is not like the normal tiredness every typical individual feels on occasion. It is a bone-weary exhaustion that drains one's body of energy and turns every activity into a chore. About 40% to 70% percent of people with fibromyalgia also have uncomfortable symptoms of irritable bowel syndrome, including:

- Stomach pain

- Gas

- Bloating

- Nausea

- Constipation and or diarrhea

About 70% of people with fibromyalgia have migraine headaches or chronic tension, which are frequently intense. Headaches may begin from painful neck, head, or shoulder muscles.

Unusual Symptoms

Below are other unusual symptoms that you might not expect; you may experience them infrequently or not at all. They do, however, occur in some people with fibromyalgia:

- Swelling

- Jaw pain

- Profuse sweating

- Chest pain

- Easy bruising

- Sensitivity to light, temperature, noise

- Bladder pain

- Food allergy symptoms like wheezing, vomiting, a stuffed nose, or diarrhea

- Urgent need to urinate

In people with fibromyalgia, there is always dysfunctionality in their brain and nerves as they overreact to or misinterpret typical pain symptoms. This may happen because of a chemical imbalance in the brain or abnormality in the dorsal root affecting the brain (central pain) sensitization. Fibromyalgia can also affect one's emotions and energy levels.

Symptoms of Fibromyalgia in Women

In a general sense, women have suffered from fibromyalgia more severely than men have. More women than men have been diagnosed with and treated for irritable bowel syndrome (IBS), morning fatigue, and widespread, chronic pain. Painful menstruation is common among women with fibromyalgia, too.

Nevertheless, when the 2016 revisions to the diagnostic criteria were put to the test, more men were diagnosed with fibromyalgia, which may lessen the degree of distinction between the level of pain men and women experience. It's important to note that the transition to menopause could make the condition worse.

Symptoms of Fibromyalgia in Men

Men get fibromyalgia, too. They may remain undiagnosed because the condition is majorly seen as a woman's illness. Current statistics show, however, that as the 2016 diagnostic protocol is applied more often, more men are being diagnosed.

Men also have intense pain and emotional symptoms from fibromyalgia. According to 2018 research, the ailment affects their productivity ranging from their quality of career, relationships, and life. Some of the stigma and difficulties in getting men diagnosed are a direct result of society's expectation that men in pain should suck it up.

Related Conditions

Apart from the conditions that trigger fibromyalgia, there are numerous other conditions associated with it. It would be helpful to bear in mind that some of these associated conditions are rheumatic conditions that affect the bones, joints, and muscles. Some of these associated conditions are as follows:

Lupus

This is a condition where the immune system mistakenly attacks healthy tissues and cells in numerous parts of the body.

Temporomandibular disorder (TMD)

This condition can cause pain in the cheeks, temples, jaw, and ears.

Ankylosing spondylitis

This is the swelling and pain in some parts of the spine.

Rheumatoid arthritis

You will notice this condition when the immune system mistakenly attacks healthy cells in the joints leading to swelling and pain.

Osteoarthritis

Here, damage to the joints causes stiffness and pain.

Possible Triggers of Fibromyalgia

Originally, people were diagnosed with fibromyalgia once they had widespread pain and tenderness in 11 out of 18 precise trigger points around their bodies. Healthcare personnel would analyze the person to detect pain by just touching or pressing these trigger points firmly.

The common trigger points include:

- Tops of the shoulders

- Hips

- Upper chest

- Knees

- Back of the head

- Outer elbows

- Back of the head

For the most part, trigger points are no longer a part of the diagnostic process. Instead, healthcare professionals may diagnose fibromyalgia if you have experienced pain in 4 out of the 5 areas of discomfort as defined by the 2016 revised diagnostic criteria.

Often, fibromyalgia is triggered by stressful events such as physical stress or psychological (emotional) stress.

Some of the possible triggers for this condition are:

- A virus-related infection

- A wound

- Having an operation

- Being in an abusive relationship

- Giving birth

- The death of a loved one

- The failure of a relationship

It is essential to note that fibromyalgia does not always develop after any noticeable trigger; sometimes, it just develops out of the blue.

In a nutshell, fibromyalgia is a long-term ailment that causes sleep disorders, depression, widespread pain, fatigue, and a host of other symptoms. At the moment, it doesn't have a cure, and researchers don't have an in-depth understanding of its causes. Men and women who have fibromyalgia experience the symptoms differently, but the possible triggers remain the same among them.

Chapter Four: How Fibromyalgia is Diagnosed

If you experience fatigue almost all the time and have muscle pains and aches, you may think you have the flu or another similar illness. If the pains and aches are accompanied by gastrointestinal (GI) distress, insomnia, or brain fog, consider booking an appointment to see a medical practitioner and discuss the possibility of this combination being fibromyalgia. Before doing so, you should be sure that you have experienced these symptoms for weeks and, perhaps, months. It is pertinent to note that fibromyalgia can occur in anyone at any age but often first strikes in middle age.

Fibromyalgia is an enduring health condition that involves widespread pain through almost all the significant parts of your body. Unfortunately, there are no imaging or lab tests available for diagnosing fibromyalgia. Instead, your physician will ask you to give detailed information about the symptoms you observe. There are a series of other diseases which have almost the same symptoms as fibromyalgia, and your doctor will likely test for some of these when diagnosing you. Among these are Lyme disease, HIV, AIDS, hypothyroidism, degenerative diseases of the spine, and certain types of cancer.

The specialist can use clinical tests to eliminate many of these aforementioned conditions to determine the precise ailment you are suffering from. Be aware that this process will likely take a lot of effort, time, and of course, money. A National Fibromyalgia and Chronic Pain Association report states that on average it takes over 5 years for a patient with fibromyalgia to get an accurate diagnosis.

Difficulties Diagnosing

It is advised you book an appointment with a rheumatologist or your family doctor to discuss your symptoms. You may also start a fibromyalgia pain log to keep track of your symptoms, note how severe the pain is, and detail the impact the pain has on your day-to-day activities. Another way you can track if you have fibromyalgia is by using the arthritis power app to check your symptoms. Then, you can share the outcome with your doctor.

Here's why fibromyalgia may be hard to diagnose:

You might be visiting the wrong doctor

While the first step you should take is to talk to a health practitioner, you may want to ask for a referral to a rheumatologist. Upon visiting a rheumatologist, you will have to carry out tests to rule out health conditions with similar symptoms to fibromyalgia.

Once you're checked for fibromyalgia, you can then see a pain management specialist who would offer customized treatments should you have chronic pain. If you are unable to see a rheumatologist, perhaps because there isn't one in your area, you can talk to your family doctor about your symptoms in detail and mention that it could be fibromyalgia. The doctor will try to diagnose it to see if they can treat the symptoms.

Your doctor might not be screening you appropriately

Here is another reason why fibromyalgia can prove challenging to diagnose: doctors invest so much time and resources in screening for diseases that could be generating all the different symptoms of fibromyalgia. They might detect an entirely different condition like irritable bowel syndrome (IBS) or depression. That is why it is essential to see a specialist in fibromyalgia.

The pain cannot be seen

The inability to perceive fibromyalgia-based pain makes it quite challenging to diagnose. That is why it is essential to give detailed information of the exact pain you feel, what spurs it up, the length of time it lasts, and what makes it feel better (if at all). Most people with fibromyalgia often experience burning sensations or tingling with pain in some regions of their body and they constantly are fatigued. Be sure to confirm if you continuously have these symptoms and how often; make a list of them and submit this list to your primary healthcare provider.

Fibromyalgia often occurs with other diseases

People can have fibromyalgia together with other diseases like osteoarthritis or inflammatory arthritis. These conditions fall under the classification of chronic pain ailment. A rheumatologist performs their job by asking related questions and doing lab or imaging tests that can help differentiate between ailments. For instance, a patient might have rheumatoid arthritis, and at the same time, fibromyalgia. Such patients may be taking drugs that help reduce inflammation, yet still feel chronic pain. Should this occur, the constant pain may be due to fibromyalgia or other related conditions instead of rheumatoid arthritis. So, if you have rheumatoid arthritis, and you think you might have fibromyalgia, as well, it would be best for you to talk to your rheumatologist about it to see if they can treat the symptoms of fatigue and general body pain, too.

Physical Test and Medical History for Diagnosing Fibromyalgia

To properly diagnose fibromyalgia, your doctor will ask you about how you feel generally. This can be about the pain you've felt in the past weeks, how often you experience fatigue, the likely causes, and whether you're constantly tired all the time.

They will also ask to know the recurring pain you feel, its severity, and sensitivity in some areas of your body.

Furthermore, your primary health caregiver should ask you about other symptoms because fibromyalgia sometimes affects humans with other unrelated health issues like anxiety, frequent urination, depression, headaches, IBS, and jaw pain from clenching. This is why it is essential to have a doctor who listens to your symptoms and can easily make connections among them.

Old and New Fibromyalgia Diagnostic Criteria

In 2010, the American College of Rheumatology created new criteria for diagnosing fibromyalgia. According to the criteria, you may have fibromyalgia if you meet the requirements below:

- If you never had any disorders that could explain your symptoms

- If you have a widespread pain index score of 7 or more and a symptom severity scale score of at least 5. Or if you have a widespread pain index score of approximately 3 to 6 and a symptom severity scale score of 9 or more.

- If you feel pain that isn't a result of another disorder

- If you experienced fibromyalgia symptoms consistently for almost 3 months

- If you have pain on both sides of your body

- If you feel chronic pain in the upper and lower part of your waist

- If you feel pain in up to at least 11 out of the possible 18 tender points

To reach these criteria, you must have pain in at least 4 of these 5 regions of your body:

- The right upper region, including the arm, jaw, or shoulder

- The left upper region, including the jaw, arm, or shoulder

- The axial region, including back, abdomen, neck, or chest

- The left lower zone, including leg, buttock, or hip

- The right lower zone, including the buttock, hip, or leg

Tender Points

In the past, physicians would check about 18 specific regions on a person's body to detect how many of them were painful when pressed or touched firmly. The tender points which occur on both sides of the body are as follows:

- Knee

- Hip bone

- Lower neck in front

- Arm near the elbow

- Edge of upper breast

- The base of the skull in the back of the head

- Back of the shoulders

- Back of the neck

- Upper outer buttock

Although counting the tender points is not generally accepted today, people with fibromyalgia typically do fulfill the tender point criteria. Although some doctors still use it, it shouldn't be the ultimate test for diagnosing fibromyalgia because you can have fibromyalgia without necessarily having pain in these tender points.

Tests for Diagnosing Fibromyalgia

As already mentioned, there is no blood test to detect FBM. Your doctor may take blood in order to screen for other ailments and rule out others including lupus, rheumatoid arthritis, and hypothyroidism, among other ailments. Nevertheless, tests including erythrocyte sedimentation rate and C-reactive protein (CRP) can help diagnose inflammation in the body, although they should be found in diseases such as rheumatoid arthritis and not FBM. So, if the outcome of your CRP tests proves low or medium, and your erythrocyte sedimentation rate tests come back as low inflammation, that might rule out other diseases and compel your physician to test you for fibromyalgia.

A recent study shows that using an advanced blood test (vibrational spectroscopy) may help detect specific protein biomarkers in the blood that distinguishes FBM from other ailments.

Imaging Tests to Diagnose Fibromyalgia

Though one can see arthritis on an X-ray, the reverse is the case for fibromyalgia. If you can identify FBM symptoms and take an imaging test, but it doesn't indicate anything, then it's more likely to be fibromyalgia.

In recent research, functional brain imaging tests in people with FBM have detected abnormal pain processing in some brain areas. Magnetic resonance spectroscopy discovered higher concentrations of the neurotransmitter glutamate in some pain-related areas in FBM patients.

Other Fibromyalgia Tests

Your doctor may run some other blood tests, including:

- Erythrocyte sedimentation rate

- Cyclic citrullinated peptide test

- Complete blood count

- Thyroid function tests

- Vitamin D

- Antinuclear antibody

- Rheumatoid factor

- Celiac serology

If there's a chance that you may be suffering from a sleep disorder, your medical practitioner may also recommend an overnight sleep study.

How Doctors Know: What Happens Next If It's FBM?

As soon as your medical practitioner has diagnosed whether you meet the criteria for FBM and ruled out other ailments, they may prescribe medical treatments and lifestyle changes to help you manage and treat fibromyalgia.

Your health caregiver may suggest some antidepressant medication that will not only treat depression but also manage the fatigue and pain associated with FBM.

Another thing your doctor can recommend for fibromyalgia is anti-seizure medications that can help with nerve-related pain, such as Lyrica (pregabalin) and Neurontin (gabapentin).

Your doctor may propose cognitive behavioral therapy and conversational therapy, massage therapy, chiropractic help, and/or acupuncture, all of which can help reduce pain and symptoms. Your physician will also likely advise you to engage in regular exercise and self-care practices.

Chapter Five: Complications of Fibromyalgia

Once you have been diagnosed with Fibromyalgia due to the signs and symptoms you have displayed, it's time to focus on getting better. As you do so, it's important for you to know that Fibromyalgia can be made worse if you're not mindful.

Common Complications

During treatment, the disease could become aggravated by some complications. Some of the complications associated with fibromyalgia are:

Increased hospitalizations

People who have fibromyalgia have higher chances of being hospitalized compared to someone living without the condition. This is because people suffering from this condition often have many accompanying health diseases. It is still not known if fibromyalgia is the cause of these related diseases or if the diseases are responsible for the development of fibromyalgia.

The following conditions are common among people living with FBM: chronic fatigue syndrome, migraines, and tension headaches. These ailments sometimes require medical attention for their treatment.

Most of the conditions that would require fibromyalgia patients to spend time in hospitals have easily identifiable symptoms and you can receive specific treatments for them from your healthcare provider. Diseases affecting the bowels are different, however, as they are harder to treat.

Increased risk of rheumatic conditions

The Centers for Disease Control and Prevention postulated that fibromyalgia patients are at a higher risk of developing rheumatic conditions. Examples of those conditions are rheumatoid arthritis, osteoarthritis, systemic lupus erythematosus, and ankylosing spondylitis. This higher risk is because FBM patients often experience joint pain and stiffness, muscle spasms, leg muscle weakness, and inflammation of the hands, feet, and limbs.

Another study published in Frontiers in Human Science also postulated that patients who have fibromyalgia might lose their ability to walk correctly and maintain balance while standing due to changes in their walking gait. Some FBM patients also find it challenging to move around due to stiffness and pain.

Depression

Many patients with fibromyalgia suffer from depression. This has led many to believe that there are biological and physiological similarities between depression and fibromyalgia. If this is true, it suggests that depression would accompany fibromyalgia or vice versa.

Studies have also shown that 90% of people battling fibromyalgia have symptoms of depression. Research has also shown that adults with fibromyalgia are over 3x more likely to experience depression than those not living with the condition. Depression that accompanies fibromyalgia often occurs due to the isolation and pain that the patient experiences when battling this disorder.

Typically, the best way to deal with depression is through therapy. One-on-one sessions with a qualified therapist are advised to help you understand your body and how your thoughts impact your health. You can also join a support group to find people suffering from similar conditions, which should help you manage the feelings that you are experiencing, such as loneliness or isolation. Depression is treatable; seek help if you feel the need.

Poor quality of life

When we are injured or experiencing pain, we always wish for the pain to end to get back to our everyday lives because pain is not an enjoyable experience. People with fibromyalgia are constantly experiencing pain, which inhibits their ability to perform many essential functions, and this directly impacts their quality of life. An example is that most people suffering from FBM find it hard to sleep for the required hours needed to fully rest and regenerate.

Some people with this disorder experience sleep apnea, which can cause daytime fatigue and increase the risk factor of suffering from conditions like heart problems, Type 2 diabetes, and liver problems. Most FBM patients are unable to function effectively at work, school, and in their homes.

The pain that fibromyalgia patients feel limits their mobility which in turn makes it very difficult for them to concentrate during daily activities. Fibro-fog is one of the symptoms that many FBM patients display. Fibro-fog is a cognitive dysfunction associated with fibromyalgia; the patients who show these symptoms are easily distracted, display short-term memory loss, have difficulty holding conversations, and experience forgetfulness.

Fibro-fog is one of the reasons why many people with FBM cannot work; those that can work are not as productive as others and it lowers the quality of life for such individuals. This symptom increases the difficulty of certain activities and makes things that were once fun tedious and stressful. The difficulty is because of the pain and fatigue that comes with the condition. Most FBM patients tend to become passive due to the pain they feel which makes them opt-out of their usual routines and social life.

Another associated factor that affects the quality of life of fibromyalgia patients is a flare-up. When the symptoms associated with fibromyalgia increase or there is an increase in the intensity of the symptoms, it is called a flare-up. Flare-ups can occur without any prior warning, but most of them happen when the patient is stressed or depressed. Some flare-ups can last for days, while others might last for weeks.

Obesity and physical deconditioning

It is common for fibromyalgia patients to experience weight gain. It could be very frustrating that you are increasing in size while battling with diverse fibromyalgia symptoms. Obesity is a common complication for several reasons.

Fibromyalgia causes changes in hormonal levels. Some of the affected hormones are insulin, and serotonin. Hormonal imbalances in the body can cause increased hunger due to slowed metabolism and fatigue. Not only does lack of sleep affect the quality of life of fibromyalgia patients, but it can lead to weight gain because such individuals have an increased appetite, reduced metabolism, and desire to eat high-energy food without the ability or desire to add physical movement to counteract the increased caloric intake.

Extreme sensitivity

A common complication in people suffering from fibromyalgia is that they become extremely sensitive to everything around them. The things they become sensitive to come from common environmental factors like light, sound, odors, perfumes, aftershave lotion, dryer sheets, and laundry detergents. Some patients also became extremely sensitive to differences in the weather like barometric pressure changes and the beginning of winter.

Many people with this condition have reported that they experience unusual skin sensitivity. Some describe the unusual sensation as feeling like a really bad sunburn. Some of the patients also noticed that the pigmentation and texture of their skin has changed.

Poor Sex Life

Many studies have shown people living with fibromyalgia have unsatisfying sex lives. The studies show that they have less desire and experience more pain; they are also less excited about things, including sex. Sex is a physical, emotional, and mental activity. People living with fibromyalgia are known to be weak physically, emotionally, and mentally due to the impact of the pain on their lives. Most of them are known to have a bad perception of their body image, which also affects their confidence to participate in sexual activities.

This chapter has shown that living with fibromyalgia could result in many complications if it is not properly managed. It is essential that all individuals living with this condition receive the best care mentally, emotionally, and physically.

Chapter Six: Treating Fibromyalgia Medically

Medical practitioners are still not sure about the causative factors of fibromyalgia, as this condition makes a person feel pain despite them lacking signs of inflammation or physical injuries. Nevertheless, there are widely accepted medical treatments that may help relieve the symptoms.

Fibromyalgia Treatment Methods

There are two ways one can treat fibromyalgia. They are:

- Self-care strategies

- Medication

The truth is, there is not a single treatment that works for all fibromyalgia. Applying multiple approaches can usually help make the biggest difference.

Medication Approach

Medication can help limit fibromyalgia pain to a reasonable extent and also improve sleep. You can make either of the following choices:

Antidepressants

Savella (milnacipran HCL) and Cymbalta (Duloxetine) may help relieve the fatigue and pain associated with fibromyalgia. Your medical practitioner may also prescribe muscle relaxants such as cyclobenzaprine or amitriptyline, which may help you sleep well and restore the correct balance to neurotransmitters.

Pain relievers

Many fibromyalgia patients have found some relief in over-the-counter pain relievers such as ibuprofen (Motrin, Advil, etc.), naproxen sodium (Aleve, etc.), or acetaminophen (Tylenol, Excedrin, etc.). It is essential to note that opioid medications are not advised because they can easily lead to dependence; additionally, opioids will often make the pain worsen as time goes on. The side effects and addiction risks are why most health providers advise patients against using narcotics to treat fibromyalgia.

Anti-seizure drugs

Medications explicitly designed to treat epilepsy are often helpful in reducing certain types of pain. Lyrica (pregabalin) was the first drug approved by the Food and Drug Administration to treat fibromyalgia, and it was developed to stop nerve cells from sending out pain signals. At the same time, on rare occasions, Gabapentin (Neurontin) can be helpful to reduce symptoms of fibromyalgia such as nerve pain. Anti-seizure drugs come with some side effects like dizziness, dry mouth, swelling, and weight gain.

Other Treatment Methods

Medical marijuana

Medical marijuana has been shown to relieve symptoms of fibromyalgia. Recent research shows that people with fibromyalgia who took medical cannabis experienced some or all of the following:

- Enhanced relaxation

- Improved mental health

- A reduction of stiffness and pain

- Feelings of well-being

- An increase in sleepiness

More research is needed, however, about the benefits of medical marijuana for fibromyalgia because it has some side effects, which include difficulty concentrating and clouded judgment.

Take Vitamin D

People with fibromyalgia usually have low levels of vitamin D. A 2013 study shows that people with fibromyalgia felt physically better and experienced less fatigue when they took vitamin D supplements.

There is still ongoing research about new methods that can be used to treat fibromyalgia medically. In this chapter, I have mentioned the medical options that can be used to alleviate the symptoms of fibromyalgia. If you are living with this condition, do not assume these are the best options for you based on what you have read. I always advise you to visit a doctor before starting your treatment. Plus, some alternatives can be used to treat the symptoms of fibromyalgia, and it's advisable to discuss these options with your doctor, too.

Chapter Seven: Alternative Fibromyalgia Therapies

Therapy Treatments for Fibromyalgia

There are several therapies one can apply to help reduce the effect of fibromyalgia on their life in general and their body in particular. Instances of such treatments include:

Counseling

Many times, people living with fibromyalgia have challenging, stressful periods that test their ability and resilience. In an earlier chapter, I mentioned that many people living with this condition are often anxious and depressed. One way to manage those risk factors is by speaking to someone who's experienced with it. That is why it is recommended to talk to a counselor. Talking with a counselor, a mental health therapist, a psychologist, or a psychiatrist can help boost your belief in your capabilities and teach you some approaches you can apply to deal with stressful situations.

Occupational Therapy

Fibromyalgia affects all nerve endings of the body, which inhibits the ability of patients to carry out everyday tasks. Occupational therapy is a treatment that helps people struggling with movement and coordination. The work of an occupational therapist is to help you adjust your work area or adjust the way you carry out specific tasks that will help reduce stress on your body.

Physical Therapy

Licensed physical therapists have a background in the study of movement. Many fibromyalgia patients struggle with daily activities, and they would benefit from stretching and strengthening programs. A physical therapist will teach you the exercises to engage in that will improve your flexibility, strength, and stamina. A physical therapist can work with people of all ages, from infants to adults. Studies conducted on the impact of physical therapy have shown that one-on-one appointments with physical therapists can help restore overall health. Physical therapy has been effective in treating fibromyalgia symptoms as they help reduce fatigue and stiffness.

Hydrotherapy

Many studies have shown that using water at different temperatures internally and externally for fibromyalgia patients can have many benefits. A physical therapist can conduct this therapy, and it can help fibromyalgia patients to use their muscles and joints without stressing them too much. The most suitable kind of hydrotherapy for treating fibromyalgia is balneotherapy. Balneotherapy involves soaking the patient in mineral-rich waters or natural mineral hot springs to alleviate pain. This therapy can be performed at home, health centers, spas, and physical therapy clinics. Hydrotherapy is very common in sports to help professional athletes recover faster and for pain alleviation. You should also know that hydrotherapy is not appropriate for everyone as it could cause skin maceration and infection. Before you use this therapy, ensure your doctor and physical therapist are aware of your specific needs.

Biofeedback

The full effectiveness of this therapy is unknown. Biofeedback aims to promote relaxation, which logically can help to relieve stress-related conditions. In a biofeedback session, electrodes and finger sensors are connected to a monitor to display light and an image that shows your blood pressure, sweating, breathing rate, skin temperature, heart rate, and muscle activity. This technique would allow you to have more control over involuntary actions that are controlled by the nervous system. The idea of biofeedback is that if you have more control over how your mind works, you will have increased control over your health. It has proved effective in treating conditions like migraines, high blood pressure, and chronic pain. It has helped fibromyalgia patients to locate tight muscles and relax them, helping to treat the symptoms associated with this condition. This therapy can be used on anyone living with FBM irrespective of their age, provided they are not suffering from other underlying conditions like heart rhythm problems. Consult your doctor before trying biofeedback.

Cognitive Behavioral Therapy (CBT)

This is another treatment approach that uses the abilities of the mind to improve the health of an individual. Cognitive behavioral therapy aims to provide ways to explore our actions and thoughts by identifying negative thoughts and behavioral patterns. Once you identify the negative thoughts that have played a part in the negative orientation of your mind and actions, you can now start learning how to channel the power in your mind into positive thoughts and actions. This is considered by many to be the best form of psychotherapy.

The ideas behind cognitive-behavioral therapy and biofeedback are similar as they both believe that emotions, actions, and thoughts are connected. For example, if you are feeling too much stress at work, and this stress has been affecting your output, you can use this therapy to make behavioral changes. There have been many publications about the effectiveness of treating fibromyalgia with cognitive behavioral therapy. This therapy has successfully reduced the level of pain experienced in patients with this condition.

Chiropractic Treatment Techniques

This treatment method is performed by chiropractors who are skilled in the art of locating the pressure points that bother fibromyalgia patients. There are many treatment regimens under chiropractic care. The treatment procedure depends on the type of condition affecting the patient. Many often confuse it with massage, but chiropractors focus on the entire musculoskeletal system while massage focuses on muscles.

Self-care Strategy

Applying a self-care approach is very crucial in the management of fibromyalgia. This approach can, at times, be critical. If you have fibromyalgia, you may consider applying the following lifestyle and home remedies to your routine.

Maintain a healthy lifestyle

Eat good food. Minimize how much caffeine you consume. Do not use tobacco products. Ensure that you do something that you find exciting and fulfilling every day.

Regular exercise

On the one hand, this may increase your pain in the short term. On the other hand, when you do it gradually and regularly, exercise will likely reduce your symptoms. Some of the appropriate exercises you can do are biking, swimming, walking, and water aerobics. Talk to a physical therapist to help you develop a home exercise program. Other regular exercises you can engage in include maintaining good posture, stretching, and relaxing. Do not underestimate the power of exercising regularly.

Sleep hygiene

Because fatigue is one of the main fibromyalgia symptoms, getting good quality sleep cannot be overemphasized. Apart from taking enough time to sleep well, ensure to practice good sleeping habits, such as allocating a specific time to go to bed, getting up at the same time every day, and reducing naps during the daytime.

Stress management

Make it a habit to avoid overexertion and emotional stress. Allot some time for yourself each day to relax and unwind. You don't have to be remorseful about this; ensure you give yourself the time it takes. Make sure to stick to the timing and do not change your routine. Always remember that people who quit doing work or drop all activities may likely do worse than those who remain active in their efforts. You can engage other stress management mechanisms like mediation or deep-breathing exercises.

Set a pace

Setting a pace for yourself will do you good. Make it a habit to keep your activity on an even level each day. If you engage yourself too much on your good days, you may have more bad days ahead. Moderation implies not doing too much on your good days and at the same time not limiting your ability or doing too little on the days the symptoms flare up.

Alternative medicine

Alternative and complementary therapies for stress and pain management are not new. People have been practicing some of these alternative therapies for centuries, including yoga and meditation. The benefits of these practices have become increasingly popular and integrated around the world in recent times, especially with people who have long-term illnesses such as fibromyalgia.

Many of these treatments appear to relieve one's stress and limit pain. Many practices remain untested because scientists haven't yet taken the time to carry out adequate research on them.

Yoga and tai chi

Yoga and tai chi exercises have proven to help regulate fibromyalgia symptoms. This regulation and relief is a result of several common strategies of yoga and tai chi: slowness, meditation, deep/mindful breathing, and overall relaxation.

Massage therapy

Massage therapy is one of the oldest health care methods and is still in practice in modern society. Massage may be helpful as it will reduce your heart rate, relax your muscles, increase your body's natural painkiller production, and improve the range of movement in your joints. In a nutshell, massage therapy often helps relieve you of stress and anxiety.

Acupuncture

Acupuncture is a Chinese medical system that involves restoring the normal balance of life forces by thrusting very fine needles through the skin to different depths. According to Western theories of acupuncture, the fine needles cause changes in blood flow and levels of neurotransmitters in the spinal cord and the brain.

Making Plans for Your Appointment

It will be okay if you recognize and remember that the signs and symptoms of fibromyalgia feel almost the same way as other disorders do. Because of this, it is wise to see your doctor before going on to receive a diagnosis. Your family physician may refer you to a specialist whose area of specialization is in the treatment of arthritis and other similar conditions like a rheumatologist.

Chapter Eight: Helping a Loved One Through Fibromyalgia

Living with someone, especially a loved one that has fibromyalgia, can be very tough, especially when they are experiencing long bouts of pain. Even though you will not feel the exact pain that the person feels, seeing someone you love in pain creates an uneasy feeling. This will no doubt impact how you live your life as you will have to help them through tough periods and be there for them when they need it, even if it is not comfortable for you.

Ways to Support a Loved One

If you want to give a helping hand to a loved one that has fibromyalgia, you have to accept the condition and all that comes with fibromyalgia. Once you have accepted what their diagnosis means, you can now start assisting, and there are many ways to be supportive of a loved one battling fibromyalgia, listed here:

Learn About Fibromyalgia

The first thing to do is to educate yourself about the condition. Many people are eager to help, but they do not know what fibromyalgia is. Lack of knowledge will severely affect your chances of helping a loved one and you could end up being more of a burden than a helper. Reading this book is a great first step!

Help them find a routine that works

In previous chapters, I have discussed many ways that can be used to manage the symptoms, and you can choose from any of them. Finding the right regime can take time because treating fibromyalgia often involves medication and physical therapy, among other alternative therapies. A good way to show support is by taking time out to discuss some of the options and taking the time to assist them in adjusting to new routines. Sometimes the people who are suffering from this condition might be reluctant to properly evaluate the options and it would be helpful to have someone who cares about them suggest possible treatment strategies.

Remind them they do not have to do much

Not only is fibromyalgia challenging physically, but it is also challenging emotionally, and many people who have this condition are left frustrated by their inability to do certain things. In those moments when they are feeling weak, support them and remind them that being unable to do some things does not make them less strong. Most of them become exhausted in an attempt to prove to themselves that they are not weak, and this stubbornness might lead to more pain.

Instead of them feeling like they have to prove anything, remind them that they just have to take care of themselves, and it is okay to stop.

Encourage them

The regime for their treatment will become challenging, especially when they are experiencing a lot of pain and fatigue. Always be there to encourage them as they need a lot of determination to keep going. For example, you can join them in the regime to motivate them or do things that you know can motivate them. You can help them to create a balance between resting and carrying out their daily regime.

The little things matter

The little things that you do for people with this condition are greatly appreciated. The willingness to help them with the little things can be used as a source of motivation when they feel weak. It also shows them that they are loved and that there is a good support system behind them.

Take time to recharge

You will not be able to give if you do not have your own support system; to be a support system for someone with fibromyalgia will take its toll on you. Before you get grumpy or become extremely frustrated with the person, take a break and come back after recharging. Many people feel that leaving, even for a short time, is abandoning the person in their time of need, but it's not. It is very okay to take time off and come back renewed.

Stay positive

Courage is not the absence of fear but the ability to move forward despite fear and overwhelming odds. Fibromyalgia is a chronic condition that is very challenging, but it is not a death sentence, and you can help manage the symptoms successfully. Do not focus on the negatives of the condition; keep in mind the fact that it can be managed. If you are supporting someone with the condition, ensure you keep a positive attitude as it will rub off on the person and inspire them.

Conclusion

You have now learned about fibromyalgia, it's signs and symptoms, diagnostic criteria, and different methods of treatment. Contrary to popular opinion, fibromyalgia is not a death sentence. We have explored the different, potential causes of this condition since anyone can be diagnosed with fibromyalgia, even though statistics point out that it is most prevalent in middle-aged individuals.

The first step in receiving treatment for fibromyalgia, is of course, being officially diagnosed with it. As you have learned, diagnosis is not always a straightforward process, and you may need to consult with multiple professionals. Be diligent, and remember not to self-diagnose, as there are several other conditions with similar symptoms to Fibromyalgia.

Once diagnosed, you will likely be prescribed with some medical treatments by your doctor, usually in the form of medication and physical therapy. With the approval of your healthcare professional, don't be afraid to also add in some additional alternative treatment methods, such as therapy, massage, acupuncture, yoga, tai chi, or meditation.

While Fibromyalgia is considered a chronic condition, remember that with treatment, symptoms are often dramatically improved, and can even go into remission.

Thank you for taking the time to read this book and learn more about Fibromyalgia – an ailment that far too many people remain uninformed about. And if you are one of the people currently suffering from fibromyalgia, I hope this book was able to help you, and I wish you the best of luck in your journey to improving your health.

Resources

"Causes: Fibromyalgia." *NHS*, 20 Feb. 2019, www.nhs.uk.
https://www.nhs.uk/conditions/fibromyalgia/causes/

Cherney, Kristeen. "Everything You Need to Know about Fibromyalgia: Fibromyalgia Risk Factors." *Healthline,* 29 June 2020, www.healthline.com.
https://www.healthline.com/health/fibromyalgia

Coleman-Williams, Frances. "7 ways to support someone with Fibromyalgia." *Metro,* 3 Feb. 2017, www.metro.co.uk.
https://metro.co.uk/2017/02/03/7-ways-to-support-someone-with-fibromyalgia-6413470/

Dellwo, Adrienne. "Living with someone who has Fibromyalgia or ME/CFS: Bridging the gap between your old life and your new one." *VeryWellHealth*, 25 Jan. 2020, www.verywellhealth.com.
https://www.verywellhealth.com/tips-for-living-with-someone-who-has-fibromyalgia-715871

Felman, Adam. "Everything you need to know about Fibromyalgia." *Medical News Today*, 5 Jan. 2018, www.medicalnewstoday.com.
https://www.medicalnewstoday.com/articles/147083

"Fibromyalgia: Diagnosis." *Mayo Clinic,* 24 Sept. 2019,
www.mayoclinic.org.
https://www.mayoclinic.org/diseases-
conditions/fibromyalgia/diagnosis-treatment/drc-
20354785

"Fibromyalgia: Symptoms and Causes." *Mayo Clinic,* 7 Oct.
2020, www.mayoclinic.org.
https://www.mayoclinic.org/diseases-
conditions/fibromyalgia/symptoms-causes/syc-20354780

"Fibromyalgia: Understand how it's diagnosed." *Mayo Clinic,*
18 Sept. 2020, www.mayoclinic.org.
https://www.mayoclinic.org/diseases-
conditions/fibromyalgia/in-depth/fibromyalgia-
symptoms/art-20045401

M, Collen, "How to Treat Fibromyalgia: Fibromyalgia and
Pain." *Healthline,* 11 March 2019, www.healthline.com.
https://www.healthline.com/health/fibromyalgia-
treatments-for-pain

"Symptoms of Fibromyalgia." *NHS,* 20 Feb. 2019, www.nhs.uk.
https://www.nhs.uk/conditions/fibromyalgia/symptoms/

Villines, Zawn, "How to Relieve Fibromyalgia Pain: Medical
Treatment." *Medical News Today,* 18 April 2018,
www.medicalnewstoday.com.

https://www.medicalnewstoday.com/articles/321534#med
ical-treatments

Watson, Stephanie. "Signs and Symptoms of Fibromyalgia:
    Main Signs and Symptoms." *Healthline,* 13 Sept. 2018,
    www.healthline.com.
    https://www.healthline.com/health/fibromyalgia/signs-of-
    fibromyalgia